# BREAST CANCER DIET PLAN AND COOKBOOK FOR NEWLY DIAGNOSED

Transform Your Health with Simple, Flavorful, and Anticancer Recipes for Breast Cancer Prevention and Total Recovery

**Eddy Beckett, MD**

representations or warranties about the completeness, accuracy, reliability, suitability, or availability of the publication or the information, products, services, or related graphics contained in the publication for any purpose. Your reliance on such material is thus entirely at your own risk.

We shall not be liable for any loss or harm, including without limitation, indirect or consequential loss or damage, or any loss or damage deriving from loss of data or profits originating from or in connection with the use of this publication.

This publication may contain links to websites that are not under our control. We have no influence on the nature, content, or accessibility of other websites. The presence of any links does not constitute a suggestion or endorsement of the ideas expressed within them.

Every effort is taken to maintain the publication operational. Nevertheless, we accept no responsibility for, and will not be accountable for, the publication being momentarily unavailable owing to technical reasons beyond our control.

# Table of Contents

# FOREWORD

Welcome to an inspiring voyage of empowerment, nourishment, and restoration as we embark on a culinary journey specifically tailored to navigate the complexities of breast cancer. This cookbook is a heartfelt testament, utilizing the transformative potential of nutrition and culinary artistry to assist individuals grappling with the challenges of breast cancer.

Contained within these pages are not merely recipes, but invaluable life lessons transcending the mere act of nourishing the body. We firmly believe that food possesses the remarkable ability to foster connections and provide the sustenance needed to persevere through adversity. Our overarching objective is to offer a comprehensive perspective on nutrition, one that not only addresses the physiological needs of the body but also acknowledges the profound psychological benefits of indulging in delicious, wholesome fare.

The battle against breast cancer is a deeply personal journey, with each individual traversing a unique path. Within this compendium, you will discover meticulously curated recipes meticulously crafted to cater to the diverse dietary requirements that may arise at different stages of treatment and recovery. From immune-boosting elixirs to comforting yet nutritious dishes, our culinary creations are designed to imbue you with the strength and optimism necessary to embrace each new day with resilience.

As you navigate through this cookbook, you'll embark on a voyage of discovery, unraveling the intricate interplay between food and health. Armed with this knowledge, you'll be empowered to make informed decisions regarding the components to incorporate into your treatment plan.

At the heart of this cookbook lies the principle of self-determination. We encourage you to embrace the transformative potential of cooking as you embark on an exploration of new ingredients, flavors, and culinary techniques. Infusing your culinary creations with intention, love, and healing energy is just as vital as following the recipes precisely.

Remember, you are not alone on this journey. This cookbook serves as a celebration of the unifying power of food and a testament to its innate healing properties. May the dishes you create within these pages provide you with comfort, strength, and inspiration as you embark on this culinary odyssey.

From our kitchen to yours, we extend our heartfelt wishes that this cookbook will not only fortify you with strength and hope but also tantalize your taste buds with an array of delectable recipes as you confront breast cancer head-on.

# CHAPTER I: What Constitutes a Breast Cancer Diet?

No single food or diet can guarantee protection from or trigger breast cancer. However, the choices we make in what we eat can influence our risk of developing breast cancer and our overall health while living with it. Breast cancer is a multifaceted condition with various factors contributing to it, some of which, like age, family history, genetics, and gender, are beyond our control.

Nevertheless, we can manage certain factors like smoking, physical activity, body weight, and diet. Research suggests that around 30–40% of all cancers could be influenced by dietary factors. What we consume directly impacts our health, including our susceptibility to complex illnesses like breast cancer.

However, applying the latest research findings to our daily lives, especially amid the stress of a cancer diagnosis, can be challenging. It's crucial to realize that no specific foods have been proven to directly prevent cancer or reduce its recurrence risk.

Instead, adopting a consistently healthy eating pattern is key. This involves consuming a plant-based, high-fiber diet while avoiding highly processed foods and overeating. Such a dietary approach is more beneficial for overall health, including lowering cancer risk, compared to rigid, hard-to-sustain diets.

One critical aspect of the diet-cancer relationship is body fat. Excess fat, especially when inflamed, can contribute to conditions like diabetes and heart disease, and cancer cells utilize this fat for energy. Our eating habits heavily influence both the quantity and quality of our fat tissue, which in turn affects cancer development.

Even if someone thought they were eating healthily before a cancer diagnosis, emerging research suggests otherwise. How we've been eating over the years can significantly impact cancer behavior and our body's response to therapy.

Healthy eating serves as an investment in our health, akin to financial savings or insurance. It can potentially improve cancer outcomes and mitigate side effects of treatment, such as mouth sores, low appetite, nausea, and vomiting. Therefore, maintaining a balanced diet is especially crucial during breast cancer treatment to aid in healing and alleviate treatment-related challenges.

# The Influence of Dietary Choices on Breast Cancer

The prevention and management of breast cancer are profoundly influenced by the dietary choices we make. Our food intake not only impacts our overall well-being but also plays a crucial role in bolstering our immune system and resilience when facing breast cancer.

Consuming a healthy, nutrient-rich diet has been demonstrated to lower the risk of developing breast cancer. Evidence suggests that incorporating a diet abundant in fruits, vegetables, whole grains, and lean proteins can mitigate this risk by shielding cells from damage induced by free radicals and oxidative stress.

Nutrition is integral in supporting individuals undergoing breast cancer therapy. Maintaining muscle mass and facilitating the healing of damaged tissues before and after treatment hinges on adequate protein intake. Nutrient-dense foods play a pivotal role in managing treatment-related side effects, boosting energy levels, and promoting overall health.

Chronic inflammation is believed to contribute to the initiation and progression of cancer. Introducing more anti-inflammatory foods such as fatty fish, nuts, seeds, and vibrant-colored vegetables into the diet may help regulate inflammation and bolster immunity. The efficiency of the immune system in identifying and eliminating abnormal cells in the body is pivotal.

The adverse effects of breast cancer therapy can impact an individual's appetite, digestion, and nutritional intake. A balanced diet can alleviate treatment-related symptoms like nausea, fatigue, and gastrointestinal issues. Incorporating soft, easily digestible foods and ensuring adequate fluid intake are imperative.

Maintaining a healthy weight is crucial in reducing the risk of breast cancer and optimizing the efficacy of therapeutic interventions. Adopting a well-rounded diet and engaging in regular physical activity can facilitate weight management and promote overall fitness.

Furthermore, dietary choices influence recovery and long-term well-being post-breast cancer therapy. A diet and lifestyle emphasizing nutritional density can contribute to long-term health, lower recurrence rates, and improved quality of life.

While nutrition plays a significant role in reducing the risk of and managing breast cancer, there is no singular food or nutrient that can prevent the disease. A comprehensive approach to breast cancer prevention and wellness encompasses various factors, including a nutritious diet, regular exercise, maintaining a healthy weight, and routine medical screenings. Seeking guidance from healthcare professionals or registered dietitians specialized in cancer nutrition can provide personalized advice and support tailored to individual needs.

# CHAPTER II: Recommendations for the Diet for Breast Cancer

The primary objective of these dietary guidelines for individuals with breast cancer is to support overall health, enhance immune function, and manage treatment-related side effects effectively. While these recommendations may not be universally applicable to all breast cancer patients, they offer valuable insights that can aid in navigating the complexities of the condition.

Opt for foods that are abundant in essential vitamins, minerals, and antioxidants, prioritizing whole, unprocessed options. The foundation of a breast cancer diet revolves around incorporating fresh produce, whole grains, lean proteins, nuts, seeds, and healthy fats. These nutrient-rich meals play a crucial role in bolstering immune defenses and facilitating the healing process.

Antioxidant-rich foods are particularly beneficial as they safeguard cells against oxidative stress. Sources of antioxidants abound in berries, citrus fruits, leafy greens, and brightly colored vegetables, offering protection and promoting cellular health.

Maintain a balanced diet that includes a diverse array of macronutrients, ensuring adequate intake of carbohydrates, proteins, and fats. Protein is indispensable for tissue repair and immune function, while complex carbohydrates and healthy fats provide sustained energy levels throughout the day.

Hydration is paramount, especially during medical therapy, to counteract dehydration. Increase fluid intake through water-rich fruits and vegetables, alongside consuming adequate amounts of water.

Incorporate ample healthy fats into your diet, such as avocados, olive oil, almonds, and fatty fish, which are rich in omega-3 fatty acids known for their anti-inflammatory properties.

High-fiber foods like whole grains, legumes, fruits, and vegetables can aid in managing common side effects like constipation associated with certain medications.

Adopt mindful cooking techniques that preserve the nutritional integrity of foods, opting for methods like steaming, baking, or sautéing over deep-frying to minimize the formation of potentially harmful compounds.

Limit consumption of processed foods, sugary snacks, and sugary beverages, as they offer minimal nutritional value and may contribute to inflammation.

Indulge in treats occasionally, but maintain a focus on nutrient-dense meals as the foundation of your diet.

Consult a registered dietitian specializing in cancer nutrition to receive personalized dietary guidance tailored to your individual needs, preferences, and treatment phase.

Recognize that the experience of breast cancer is unique to each individual, and dietary adjustments should be made in accordance with your specific symptoms, treatment regimen, and overall well-being.

Listen to your body's signals and adjust your diet accordingly, experimenting with new foods and making modifications as needed.

These recommendations serve as a starting point for developing a personalized breast cancer diet in collaboration with healthcare professionals, empowering you to make informed choices that promote health and recovery.

**Alternative Healing Methods**

The interest in integrating complementary therapies with conventional medical approaches for breast cancer treatment has been steadily increasing. These complementary therapies aim to enhance overall health, alleviate symptoms, and enhance the quality of life when utilized alongside standard medical care. While some individuals may find benefit from these adjunctive treatments, it's imperative to underscore the necessity of consulting with a medical professional before incorporating any new therapies.

Mind-body practices such as meditation, mindfulness, and yoga have garnered attention for their potential to mitigate stress, anxiety, and improve mental well-being. Given the myriad of emotional responses that a breast cancer diagnosis and treatment can evoke, these practices serve as valuable tools for managing such sentiments effectively.

Acupuncture involves the insertion of thin needles into specific points on the body and has demonstrated efficacy in alleviating treatment-related side effects like nausea, pain, and fatigue in select patients.

Massage therapy offers relaxation and relief for sore muscles, with some breast cancer patients reporting decreased treatment-related discomfort and heightened relaxation following gentle massage sessions.

Nutritional supplements and vitamins are areas of interest for individuals seeking to enhance their well-being during breast cancer treatment. However, it's essential to consult with a healthcare provider as certain supplements may interact with medications and impact treatment outcomes.

Aromatherapy utilizes essential oils to promote relaxation and soothe the mind, exhibiting potential benefits in reducing anxiety, improving sleep quality, and mitigating medication side effects for some individuals.

Engaging in creative activities such as art-making or music listening can serve as therapeutic outlets for expressing emotions and reclaiming a sense of control amidst the challenges of breast cancer treatment.

Physical activity tailored to one's fitness level can enhance strength, alleviate fatigue, and elevate mood. It's imperative to seek guidance from healthcare professionals, particularly during treatment, to ensure safety and efficacy.

Nutritional counseling can provide valuable guidance in maintaining a well-balanced diet to support overall health and potentially mitigate treatment side effects while bolstering immunity.

Access to counseling and support groups can be immensely beneficial for individuals navigating the emotional complexities of breast cancer, offering a space for sharing experiences, struggles, and triumphs, thereby fostering a sense of community and support.

Energy-based therapies such as Reiki and Healing Touch are employed to reduce stress and promote wellness, although scientific evidence supporting their efficacy remains inconclusive.

Complementary therapies should be viewed not as substitutes for conventional medical care but as adjuncts to promote holistic well-being and symptom alleviation. Given the potential risks and interactions with medical treatments, an open dialogue with healthcare professionals is essential to explore personalized options effectively. Integrating standard medical care with tailored complementary therapies can lead to a more holistic and supportive breast cancer experience.

## Integrating Mind-Body Techniques

Incorporating mind-body practices into the breast cancer journey serves as a transformative approach to enhance overall well-being and navigate the complexities of diagnosis, treatment, and recovery with greater resilience. Recognizing the intricate connection between the mind, emotions, and body, these practices offer invaluable tools for cultivating inner calm, managing stress, and fortifying emotional and psychological strength. Here's a comprehensive guide on integrating these strategies into a breast cancer diet:

Mindfulness, a practice of nonjudgmental awareness and complete presence in the moment, lies at the core of mind-body practices. Central to mindfulness is the practice of meditation, which involves directing one's attention to the breath or mental imagery. Incorporating daily mindfulness and meditation routines can be instrumental in alleviating stress and anxiety commonly experienced following a breast cancer diagnosis, offering individuals a sanctuary to cultivate inner peace amidst adversity.

Yoga, a holistic discipline encompassing physical postures, breathing exercises, and meditation, emerges as a powerful ally in promoting physical, mental, and emotional well-being for breast cancer patients. Gentle and restorative yoga practices can alleviate physical discomfort while nurturing mental clarity and emotional resilience. Moreover, yoga's adaptability allows for its integration into therapy and rehabilitation programs tailored to individual needs.

Breathwork techniques such as deep breathing and diaphragmatic breathing offer effective means to mitigate stress, anxiety, and promote relaxation. Mastery of breath control empowers individuals to navigate emotional fluctuations and foster inner tranquility amidst life's challenges.

Harnessing the power of positive affirmations and visualization techniques can facilitate the healing process by instilling hope, resilience, and mental clarity. Positive affirmations serve as uplifting mantras, while visualization cultivates a sense of optimism and envisages a successful outcome, bolstering emotional well-being.

Engaging in creative endeavors like painting, sketching, or writing serves as a therapeutic outlet to express emotions and foster self-discovery. Artistic pursuits provide avenues for emotional release, stress relief, and reconnecting with one's authentic self.

Sound therapy, utilizing instruments such as Tibetan singing bowls, offers a soothing and uplifting auditory experience that promotes relaxation and reduces stress. These melodic practices have demonstrated efficacy in enhancing calmness and mental well-being.

Mindful eating, an extension of mindfulness, emphasizes the importance of being fully present and appreciative of each bite. Adopting a mindful approach to eating enhances satisfaction, digestion, and body image, nurturing a harmonious relationship with food and body.

By incorporating these mind-body activities into the breast cancer journey, individuals can bolster mental well-being and optimize the physical aspects of therapy and recovery. These practices serve as a versatile toolkit for navigating the emotional and psychological challenges inherent in a breast cancer diagnosis and treatment. However, it is essential to introduce mind-body activities gradually and consult healthcare specialists to ensure suitability and safety. Through the adoption of these transformative techniques, individuals equip themselves with the resilience and resources needed to confront adversity and emerge stronger on the path to healing.

# CHAPTER III: Your Approach to Diet During Cancer Treatment

Medical professionals should grasp the unique needs of each patient, encompassing both medical and personal aspects. For instance, certain breast cancer tumors exhibit genetic mutations that call for targeted therapies. While these treatments may impact metabolism and insulin usage, potentially leading to weight gain, we aim to preempt this by adjusting the patient's diet beforehand.

Moreover, considering personal aspirations during cancer treatment is crucial. Some patients express a desire to shed weight for significant life events like weddings. In such cases, we adopt a gradual and safe weight loss approach, as rapid weight reduction isn't advisable.

Understanding a patient's lifestyle is paramount. Factors such as dietary habits, level of physical activity (including daily chores or childcare), and overall energy balance provide invaluable insights for tailored treatment plans.

Maintaining a balanced diet is particularly vital for individuals with breast cancer. Proper nutrition supports the body's recovery from treatment-related side effects like mouth sores, decreased appetite, nausea, and vomiting. A wholesome diet can help in various ways:

- Maintaining a healthy body weight

- Preserving tissue health

- Alleviating cancer symptoms and treatment side effects

- Strengthening the immune system

- Sustaining strength and reducing fatigue

- Enhancing overall quality of life

**Foods to Eat on the Breast Cancer Diet**

Here's a breakdown of beneficial and harmful foods concerning breast cancer:

- A variety of fruits and vegetables, including salads

- Fiber-rich foods like whole grains, beans, and legumes

- Low-fat dairy products

- Soybean-based products

- Foods abundant in vitamin D and other essential vitamins

- Anti-inflammatory foods, particularly spices

- Antioxidant-rich foods, primarily plant-based options

**Foods to Avoid on the Breast Cancer Diet**

- Alcohol

- Added sugars

- High-fat foods

- Red meat

- Processed foods

## Methods of Cooking for Breast Cancer Diet

The cooking methods used to prepare meals for a breast cancer diet have a major impact on not just the food's nutritional value but also how much the dieter enjoys eating it. Choosing appropriate cooking methods can help maintain vital nutrients while producing tasty, digestible, and health-promoting meals.

Steaming is a low-heat cooking method that helps preserve foods' original aromas, hues, and nutritional value. Vegetables benefit greatly from it since their texture and nutrient content may be maintained without the addition of lipids.

Using a tiny amount of oil and medium heat, meals are cooked rapidly in a sauté. Using this method, you may boost the flavor of your food without using too much oil. Oils that are good for your heart, like olive oil, may be used to enhance the flavor of a meal without overpowering it.

Cooking a wide variety of items, from proteins to vegetables and grains, may be accomplished through baking and roasting. These methods improve the inherent tastes and provide a pleasant texture with very little fat.

Poaching is a method of cooking in which food is slowly simmered in a liquid (usually water or broth). For delicate foods like fish and poultry, this approach is ideal since it helps to keep moisture and softness without adding additional fats.

Grilling gives meals a smokey taste without adding extra fat. Charred or burnt areas of meats may include substances that are not optimum for health, therefore it's crucial to reduce charring and avoid overcooking while grilling.

Cooking food in small bits over high heat while continually stirring is known as stir-frying, a fast and efficient cooking method. It's a great method for cooking low-fat meats and veggies without losing their brilliant colors or textures.

To slow cook, items are simmered at a low temperature for a long time. Easy-to-digest and flavorful stews, soups, and lentils may be prepared quickly and easily with this approach.

Briefly boiling meals and then plunging them into freezing water to stop the cooking process is called blanching. Useful for vegetables and fruits destined for salads or other meals, this method can help retain colors, tastes, and nutrients.

Infusing taste with herbs and spices instead of depending just on salt and fat to enhance a dish's taste, try infusing it with fresh herbs and fragrant spices. Trying out new flavor combinations is a great way to spice up your culinary routine.

The goal of the breast cancer diet is to provide the patient with nutritiously sound, yet satisfying and comfortable, meals. Using these methods, you may prepare meals that include a balanced combination of flavor, texture, and nutrition, enhancing your culinary experience with an eye toward health.

# CHAPTER IV: BREAST CANCER DIET RECIPES IDEAS

## BREAST CANCER BREAKFAST RECIPES

Quinoa Breakfast Bowl with Roasted Vegetables:

**Ingredients**

1/2 cup cooked quinoa

Assorted roasted vegetables (e.g., sweet potatoes, zucchini, bell peppers)

1 poached or fried egg (optional)

**How To Prepare**

Cook the quinoa according to package instructions and set aside.

Roast the vegetables in the oven with a drizzle of olive oil and your favorite seasonings until tender.

In a bowl, layer the cooked quinoa and roasted vegetables.

If desired, add a poached or fried egg on top for extra protein and flavor.

**Whole-Grain Cereal with Low-Fat Milk and Sliced Almonds:**

**Ingredients**

1 cup whole-grain cereal of your choice

1 cup low-fat milk (dairy or plant-based)

2 tablespoons sliced almonds


**How To Prepare**

Pour the whole-grain cereal into a bowl.

Add the low-fat milk over the cereal.

Sprinkle sliced almonds on top.

Mix the ingredients and enjoy a simple yet nutritious breakfast.

**Cottage Cheese with Peaches and a Sprinkle of Cinnamon:**

## Ingredients

1/2 cup low-fat cottage cheese

1 ripe peach, sliced

A pinch of ground cinnamon

## How To Prepare

In a bowl, spoon the low-fat cottage cheese.

Top it with sliced peaches.

Sprinkle ground cinnamon on top for added flavor.

Enjoy a light and refreshing breakfast option.

**Veggie Omelette with Tomatoes, Peppers, and Spinach:**

**Ingredients**

3 large eggs

1/4 cup diced tomatoes

1/4 cup diced bell peppers (any color)

1/2 cup fresh spinach leaves

Salt and pepper to taste

1 tablespoon olive oil

**How To Prepare**

**In a bowl, whisk the eggs and season with salt and pepper.**

**Heat olive oil in a non-stick skillet over medium heat.**

**Add the diced tomatoes and bell peppers,** sautéing until softened.

Add the fresh spinach leaves and cook until wilted.

Pour the whisked eggs over the vegetables and cook until the omelette is set.

Fold the omelette in half and serve it hot.

**Greek Yogurt with Honey and Sliced Fruits:**

**Ingredients**

1/2 cup Greek yogurt

1 tablespoon honey

Assorted sliced fruits (e.g., banana, kiwi, strawberries)

**How To Prepare**

In a bowl, spoon the Greek yogurt.

Drizzle honey over the yogurt.

Add the sliced fruits on top of the yogurt and honey.

Mix everything together or enjoy the layers as you eat.

**Oatmeal with Berries and Nuts:**

**Ingredients**

1/2 cup rolled oats

1 cup water or milk (dairy or plant-based)

1/4 cup mixed berries (blueberries, raspberries, strawberries)

1 tablespoon chopped nuts (almonds, walnuts, or your choice)

**How To Prepare**

In a saucepan, bring the water or milk to a boil.

Add the rolled oats and reduce the heat to low, simmering for about 5 minutes, or until the oats are cooked and creamy.

Transfer the oatmeal to a bowl and top with the mixed berries and chopped nuts.

Enjoy a nutritious and filling breakfast.

**Chia Seed Pudding with Fresh Mango:**

**Ingredients**

3 tablespoons chia seeds

1 cup almond milk or any milk of your choice

1 tablespoon honey or maple syrup

1 ripe mango, diced

**How To Prepare**

In a bowl, mix the chia seeds, almond milk, and honey or maple syrup.

Stir well and let it sit for 5 minutes. Stir again to avoid clumps.

Cover the bowl and refrigerate overnight or for at least 4 hours, until the mixture thickens and forms a pudding-like consistency.

Top the chia seed pudding with diced fresh mango before serving.

**Buckwheat Pancakes with Blueberries and Greek Yogurt:**

**Ingredients**

1 cup buckwheat flour

1 tablespoon honey or maple syrup

1 teaspoon baking powder

1 cup milk (dairy or plant-based)

1 large egg

1/2 cup fresh blueberries

Greek yogurt for topping

**How To Prepare**

In a mixing bowl, combine the buckwheat flour, honey or maple syrup, and baking powder.

Add the milk and egg, stirring until a smooth batter forms.

Gently fold in the fresh blueberries.

Heat a non-stick pan over medium heat and lightly grease it.

Pour 1/4 cup of the pancake batter onto the pan for each pancake.

Cook until bubbles form on the surface, then flip and cook until golden brown on both sides.

Top the pancakes with Greek yogurt and additional blueberries before serving.

**Whole-Grain Toast with Avocado and Poached Eggs:**

**Ingredients**

2 slices of whole-grain bread

1 ripe avocado

2 poached eggs

Salt and pepper to taste

**How To Prepare**

Toast the slices of whole-grain bread until they are golden brown.

Mash the avocado with a fork and spread it evenly on the toast.

Prepare poached eggs by bringing a pot of water to a simmer, adding a splash of vinegar, and gently cracking the eggs into the water. Cook for about 3-4 minutes until the whites are set.

Carefully place the poached eggs on top of the avocado toast.

Sprinkle with salt and pepper to taste.

**Sliced Apple with Almond Butter:**

**Ingredients**

1 apple, thinly sliced

2 tablespoons almond butter


**How To Prepare**

Wash and slice the apple into thin rounds or wedges.

Spread almond butter on each slice or use it as a dip for the apple slices.

Enjoy this easy and nutritious on-the-go breakfast.


**Smoothie with Spinach, Banana, and Almond Milk:**


**Ingredients**

1 cup fresh spinach leaves

1 ripe banana

1 cup unsweetened almond milk

Ice cubes (optional)

**How To Prepare**

In a blender, combine the spinach, banana, and almond milk.

Blend until smooth and creamy.

Add ice cubes if desired and blend again.

Pour the smoothie into a glass and enjoy its refreshing goodness.

## Flaxseed Granola with Soy Milk and Raspberries:

### Ingredients

1 cup flaxseed granola (store-bought or homemade)

1 cup soy milk (or any milk of your choice)

Fresh raspberries for topping

### How To Prepare

In a bowl, pour the soy milk over the flaxseed granola.

Top with fresh raspberries.

Let it sit for a few minutes to allow the granola to soften slightly.

Stir and enjoy this crunchy and nutritious breakfast.


**Brown Rice Porridge with Coconut Milk and Strawberries:**


**Ingredients**

1 cup cooked brown rice

1 cup coconut milk (canned or carton)

1 tablespoon honey or maple syrup

Sliced strawberries for topping


**How To Prepare**

In a saucepan, warm the cooked brown rice with coconut milk over low heat.

Stir in honey or maple syrup for sweetness.

Cook until the mixture thickens to a porridge-like consistency.

Transfer the brown rice porridge to a bowl and top with sliced strawberries.

**Breakfast Burrito with Black Beans, Salsa, and Avocado:**

**Ingredients**

1 large whole-grain tortilla

1/2 cup black beans (canned or cooked)

2 tablespoons salsa

1/2 avocado, sliced

1 scrambled egg (optional)

## How To Prepare

Warm the tortilla in a skillet or microwave to make it more pliable.

Spread the black beans and salsa in the center of the tortilla.

Add the sliced avocado and scrambled egg if desired.

Fold the sides of the tortilla over the fillings and roll it up into a burrito.

Serve and enjoy a hearty and flavorful breakfast.

## Green Tea with Whole-Grain Crackers and Cottage Cheese:

### Ingredients

1 cup green tea (brewed)

Whole-grain crackers

1/2 cup low-fat cottage cheese

### How To Prepare

Brew a cup of green tea following the package instructions.

Serve the green tea with a side of whole-grain crackers and a scoop of low-fat cottage cheese.

This light and balanced breakfast is perfect for a busy morning.

# BREAST CANCER LUNCH RECIPES

**Whole Wheat Wrap with Hummus, Roasted Vegetables, and Spinach:**

## Ingredients

1 whole wheat wrap or tortilla

2 tablespoons hummus

Assorted roasted vegetables (bell peppers, zucchini, eggplant, etc.)

Handful of fresh spinach leaves

## How To Prepare

Lay the whole wheat wrap on a clean surface.

Spread hummus evenly on the wrap.

Place the roasted vegetables and fresh spinach leaves on top of the hummus.

Roll the wrap tightly to form a delicious and nutritious wrap.


**Tofu and Vegetable Stir-Fry with Brown Rice:**


**Ingredients**

1 cup cubed tofu

1 cup mixed vegetables (bell peppers, broccoli, carrots, snap peas, etc.)

2 tablespoons low-sodium soy sauce

1 tablespoon hoisin sauce

1 tablespoon vegetable oil

1 clove garlic (minced)

1/2 teaspoon grated ginger

## How To Prepare

In a large skillet or wok, heat vegetable oil over medium-high heat.

Add minced garlic and grated ginger, sautéing for a minute until fragrant.

Add the cubed tofu and stir-fry until it becomes lightly browned.

Toss in the mixed vegetables and continue stir-frying until they are tender-crisp.

Mix in low-sodium soy sauce and hoisin sauce, ensuring everything is coated with the sauce.

Serve the tofu and vegetable stir-fry over cooked brown rice.

**Quinoa and Vegetable Stir-Fry:**

**Ingredients**

1 cup cooked quinoa

1 cup mixed vegetables (bell peppers, broccoli, carrots, snap peas, etc.)

2 tablespoons low-sodium soy sauce

1 tablespoon sesame oil

1 clove garlic (minced)

1/2 teaspoon grated ginger

Crushed red pepper flakes (optional for added heat)

**How To Prepare**

Heat sesame oil in a large skillet or wok over medium-high heat.

Add minced garlic and grated ginger, sautéing for a minute until fragrant.

Add the mixed vegetables to the skillet and stir-fry until they are tender-crisp.

Stir in the cooked quinoa and low-sodium soy sauce, tossing everything together until well combined.

Optionally, add crushed red pepper flakes for added spice.

Serve the quinoa and vegetable stir-fry hot.

**Baked Salmon with Steamed Broccoli and Brown Rice:**

**Ingredients**

4 ounces salmon fillet

1 cup steamed broccoli florets

1/2 cup cooked brown rice

Lemon wedges for garnish

Fresh dill (optional for garnish)

Salt and pepper to taste

**How To Prepare**

Preheat the oven to 375°F (190°C).

Season the salmon fillet with salt and pepper.

Bake the salmon in the preheated oven for about 15-20 minutes or until it's cooked through.

Steam the broccoli until tender-crisp.

Serve the baked salmon alongside steamed broccoli and cooked brown rice.

Garnish with lemon wedges and fresh dill, if desired.

**Spinach and Chickpea Salad with Lemon-Tahini Dressing:**

**Ingredients**

2 cups baby spinach leaves

1 cup cooked chickpeas

1/4 cup cherry tomatoes (halved)

2 tablespoons tahini

Juice of half a lemon

1 clove garlic (minced)

2 tablespoons water

Salt and pepper to taste

**How To Prepare**

In a large bowl, combine baby spinach, cooked chickpeas, and halved cherry tomatoes.

In a separate small bowl, whisk together tahini, lemon juice, minced garlic, water, salt, and pepper to make the dressing.

Pour the lemon-tahini dressing over the salad and toss gently to coat.

Enjoy this nutritious and flavorful salad.

## Turkey and Avocado Sandwich on Whole Grain Bread:

### Ingredients

2 slices whole grain bread

4 ounces sliced turkey breast

1/2 ripe avocado (sliced)

1 tablespoon Dijon mustard

Handful of baby spinach leaves

Salt and pepper to taste

**How To Prepare**

Lay the slices of whole grain bread on a clean surface.

Spread Dijon mustard on one side of each slice.

Layer the sliced turkey, avocado, and baby spinach on one slice of bread.

Season with salt and pepper to taste.

Top with the other slice of bread to complete the sandwich.

Cut the sandwich in half if desired, and enjoy this satisfying and nourishing lunch option.

**Lentil and Vegetable Soup:**

**Ingredients**

1 cup cooked lentils

2 cups vegetable broth

1 cup mixed vegetables (carrots, celery, onions, etc.)

1 teaspoon olive oil

1/2 teaspoon dried thyme

Salt and pepper to taste

**How To Prepare**

In a pot, heat olive oil over medium heat and sauté the mixed vegetables until softened.

Add the vegetable broth, cooked lentils, dried thyme, salt, and pepper to the pot.

Bring the soup to a simmer and cook for about 15 minutes to let the flavors meld together.

Adjust seasoning to taste.

Serve the warm and hearty lentil and vegetable soup.

**Zucchini Noodles with Tomato Sauce and Grilled Chicken:**

**Ingredients**

1 large zucchini (spiralized into noodles)

1 cup tomato sauce (homemade or store-bought)

4 ounces grilled chicken breast (cooked and sliced)

Fresh basil leaves for garnish

Grated Parmesan cheese (optional)

## How To Prepare

In a large skillet, heat the tomato sauce over medium heat until warmed through.

Add the zucchini noodles to the skillet and cook for a few minutes until they soften slightly.

Arrange the zucchini noodles on a plate and top with sliced grilled chicken.

Garnish with fresh basil leaves and grated Parmesan cheese if desired.

## Grilled Chicken Salad with Mixed Greens and Berries:

### Ingredients

4 ounces grilled chicken breast (cooked and sliced)

2 cups mixed greens (spinach, arugula, lettuce, etc.)

1/2 cup mixed berries (blueberries, strawberries, raspberries)

2 tablespoons balsamic vinaigrette dressing

### How To Prepare

In a large bowl, toss the mixed greens with the balsamic vinaigrette dressing until well coated.

Top the salad with grilled chicken slices and mixed berries.

Enjoy a refreshing and protein-packed salad.

**Vegetable and Lentil Curry with Brown Rice:**

**Ingredients**

1 cup cooked brown rice

1 cup mixed vegetables (carrots, cauliflower, peas, etc.)

1 cup cooked green lentils

1 tablespoon curry powder

1 can (14 ounces) coconut milk

1 tablespoon vegetable oil

Fresh cilantro for garnish

Salt and pepper to taste

## How To Prepare

In a large pot or skillet, heat vegetable oil over medium heat.

Add the mixed vegetables and sauté until they begin to soften.

Stir in the cooked green lentils and curry powder, coating everything evenly.

Pour in the coconut milk and simmer for a few minutes until the flavors meld together.

Season with salt and pepper to taste.

Serve the vegetable and lentil curry over cooked brown rice.

Garnish with fresh cilantro for added freshness.

## Mediterranean Salad with Feta Cheese and Olives:

**Ingredients**

2 cups mixed greens (romaine lettuce, cucumber, red onion, etc.)

1/4 cup crumbled feta cheese

1/4 cup kalamata olives

2 tablespoons extra-virgin olive oil

1 tablespoon red wine vinegar

1/2 teaspoon dried oregano

Salt and pepper to taste

## How To Prepare

In a large bowl, combine mixed greens, crumbled feta cheese, and kalamata olives.

In a separate small bowl, whisk together extra-virgin olive oil, red wine vinegar, dried oregano, salt, and pepper to make the dressing.

Drizzle the dressing over the salad and toss gently to combine.

Enjoy this refreshing and flavorsome Mediterranean-inspired salad.


## Sushi Roll with Fresh Fish and Avocado:


## Ingredients

Nori seaweed sheets

Sushi rice (cooked and seasoned with rice vinegar, sugar, and salt)

Assorted sushi-grade fish (salmon, tuna, etc.)

Avocado slices

Soy sauce and pickled ginger for dipping

**How To Prepare**

Lay a sheet of nori seaweed on a bamboo sushi rolling mat.

Spread a thin layer of sushi rice over the nori, leaving a small border around the edges.

Place slices of fresh fish and avocado in the center of the rice.

Carefully roll the sushi using the bamboo mat, applying gentle pressure to create a tight roll.

Slice the sushi roll into bite-sized pieces with a sharp knife.

Serve with soy sauce and pickled ginger for dipping.

**Quinoa Stuffed Bell Peppers:**

**Ingredients**

4 large bell peppers (any color)

1 cup cooked quinoa

1 cup cooked black beans

1 cup diced tomatoes

1/2 cup diced red onion

1/2 cup corn kernels (fresh or frozen)

1 tablespoon olive oil

1 teaspoon ground cumin

Salt and pepper to taste

Grated cheese (optional for topping)

## How To Prepare

Preheat the oven to 375°F (190°C).

Cut the tops off the bell peppers and remove the seeds and membranes.

In a large skillet, heat olive oil over medium heat.

Sauté the diced red onion until softened.

Add the cooked quinoa, black beans, diced tomatoes, and corn to the skillet, stirring to combine.

Season with ground cumin, salt, and pepper to taste.

Stuff the mixture into the bell peppers.

Optionally, sprinkle grated cheese on top of the stuffed peppers.

Place the stuffed peppers in a baking dish and bake in the preheated oven for about 25-30 minutes or until the peppers are tender and the filling is heated through.

# Grilled Shrimp and Vegetable Skewers with Quinoa:

## Ingredients

8-10 large shrimp (peeled and deveined)

Assorted vegetables (bell peppers, cherry tomatoes, zucchini, etc.)

2 tablespoons olive oil

1 tablespoon lemon juice

1 clove garlic (minced)

Fresh parsley for garnish

Cooked quinoa for serving

## How To Prepare

In a bowl, combine olive oil, lemon juice, and minced garlic to make the marinade.

Thread the shrimp and assorted vegetables onto skewers.

Brush the skewers with the marinade and let them sit for a few minutes.

Grill the skewers on medium-high heat for a few minutes on each side until the shrimp are cooked and the vegetables are charred and tender.

Serve the grilled shrimp and vegetable skewers over cooked quinoa.

Garnish with fresh parsley for added flavor.

**Chickpea and Avocado Salad with Cilantro-Lime Dressing:**

**Ingredients**

1 can (14 ounces) chickpeas (drained and rinsed)

1 ripe avocado (diced)

1 cup cherry tomatoes (halved)

1/4 cup diced red onion

Handful of fresh cilantro leaves

2 tablespoons olive oil

Juice of 1 lime

Salt and pepper to taste

**How To Prepare**

In a large bowl, combine chickpeas, diced avocado, halved cherry tomatoes, diced red onion, and fresh cilantro leaves.

In a separate small bowl, whisk together olive oil, lime juice, salt, and pepper to make the dressing.

Drizzle the cilantro-lime dressing over the salad and toss gently to coat.

This chickpea and avocado salad is light, filling, and packed with nutritious ingredients.

# BREAST CANCER DINNER RECIPES

**Quinoa Stuffed Bell Peppers:**

**Ingredients**

4 large bell peppers (any color)

1 cup cooked quinoa

1 cup cooked black beans

1 cup diced tomatoes

1/2 cup diced red onion

1/2 cup corn kernels (fresh or frozen)

1 tablespoon olive oil

1 teaspoon ground cumin

Salt and pepper to taste

Grated cheese (optional for topping)

**How To Prepare**

Preheat the oven to 375°F (190°C).

Cut the tops off the bell peppers and remove the seeds and membranes.

In a large skillet, heat olive oil over medium heat.

Sauté the diced red onion until softened.

Add the cooked quinoa, black beans, diced tomatoes, and corn to the skillet, stirring to combine.

Season with ground cumin, salt, and pepper to taste.

Stuff the mixture into the bell peppers.

Optionally, sprinkle grated cheese on top of the stuffed peppers.

Place the stuffed peppers in a baking dish and bake in the preheated oven for about 25-30 minutes or until the peppers are tender and the filling is heated through.

**Spaghetti Squash with Marinara Sauce and Turkey Meatballs:**

**Ingredients**

1 spaghetti squash

1 cup marinara sauce (homemade or store-bought)

4-6 turkey meatballs (cooked)

Fresh basil for garnish

Grated Parmesan cheese (optional for topping)

**How To Prepare**

Preheat the oven to 400°F (200°C).

Cut the spaghetti squash in half lengthwise and scoop out the seeds.

Place the squash halves cut-side down on a baking sheet lined with parchment paper.

Roast the spaghetti squash in the preheated oven for about 30-40 minutes or until the flesh is tender and easily scraped with a fork to form spaghetti-like strands.

In a saucepan, heat the marinara sauce and turkey meatballs until warmed through.

Scrape the spaghetti squash strands onto plates and top with the marinara sauce and turkey meatballs.

Garnish with fresh basil and optionally, sprinkle grated Parmesan cheese on top.

**Grilled Chicken with Roasted Vegetables:**

**Ingredients**

4 boneless, skinless chicken breasts

2 cups mixed vegetables (bell peppers, zucchini, carrots, etc.)

2 tablespoons olive oil

1 teaspoon dried herbs (rosemary, thyme, or your choice)

Salt and pepper to taste

**How To Prepare**

Preheat the grill to medium-high heat.

Season the chicken breasts with dried herbs, salt, and pepper.

In a bowl, toss the mixed vegetables with olive oil, salt, and pepper.

Grill the chicken for about 5-6 minutes per side until cooked through.

At the same time, roast the mixed vegetables in the oven at 400°F (200°C) for about 20-25 minutes until tender.

Serve the grilled chicken with the roasted vegetables.

## Grilled Shrimp with Quinoa Salad:

**Ingredients**

8-10 large shrimp (peeled and deveined)

1 cup cooked quinoa

1 cup diced cucumber

1 cup halved cherry tomatoes

1/4 cup diced red onion

2 tablespoons chopped fresh parsley

2 tablespoons lemon juice

2 tablespoons olive oil

Salt and pepper to taste

**How To Prepare**

Preheat the grill to medium-high heat.

Season the shrimp with salt and pepper.

Grill the shrimp for about 2-3 minutes on each side until they are cooked through and pink.

In a large bowl, combine cooked quinoa, diced cucumber, halved cherry tomatoes, diced red onion, and chopped fresh parsley.

In a separate small bowl, whisk together lemon juice, olive oil, salt, and pepper to make the dressing.

Pour the dressing over the quinoa salad and toss gently to coat.

Serve the grilled shrimp over the quinoa salad.

Baked Cod with Lemon-Dill Sauce and Asparagus:

**Ingredients**

4 cod fillets

1 bunch of asparagus

2 tablespoons olive oil

2 tablespoons fresh lemon juice

1 tablespoon chopped fresh dill

1 clove garlic (minced)

Salt and pepper to taste

**How To Prepare**

Preheat the oven to 400°F (200°C).

Place the cod fillets and asparagus on a baking sheet lined with parchment paper.

Drizzle olive oil and lemon juice over the cod fillets and asparagus.

Sprinkle with chopped fresh dill and minced garlic.

Season with salt and pepper to taste.

Bake in the preheated oven for about 15-20 minutes or until the cod is flaky and the asparagus is tender.

Serve the baked cod with lemon-dill sauce alongside the asparagus.

**Tofu Stir-Fry with Brown Rice:**

**Ingredients**

1 cup cubed tofu

2 cups mixed vegetables (bell peppers, broccoli, snap peas, etc.)

2 tablespoons low-sodium soy sauce

1 tablespoon hoisin sauce

1 tablespoon vegetable oil

1 clove garlic (minced)

1/2 teaspoon grated ginger

Crushed red pepper flakes (optional for added heat)

1 cup cooked brown rice

## How To Prepare

In a large skillet or wok, heat vegetable oil over medium-high heat.

Add minced garlic and grated ginger, sautéing for a minute until fragrant.

Add the cubed tofu and stir-fry until it becomes lightly browned.

Toss in the mixed vegetables and continue stir-frying until they are tender-crisp.

Mix in low-sodium soy sauce and hoisin sauce, ensuring everything is coated with the sauce.

Optionally, add crushed red pepper flakes for added spice.

Serve the tofu stir-fry over cooked brown rice.

**Chickpea and Spinach Coconut Curry:**

**Ingredients**

1 can (14 ounces) chickpeas (drained and rinsed)

2 cups fresh spinach leaves

1 can (14 ounces) coconut milk

1 tablespoon curry powder

1 tablespoon vegetable oil

1 small onion (chopped)

2 cloves garlic (minced)

1 teaspoon grated ginger

Salt and pepper to taste

Cooked basmati rice for serving

## How To Prepare

In a large skillet or pot, heat vegetable oil over medium heat.

Add chopped onion, minced garlic, and grated ginger, sautéing until the onion becomes translucent.

Stir in the chickpeas and curry powder, coating everything evenly.

Pour in the coconut milk and let it simmer for about 5 minutes to allow the flavors to meld together.

Add the fresh spinach leaves and cook until they wilt.

Season with salt and pepper to taste.

Serve the chickpea and spinach coconut curry over cooked basmati rice.

## Turkey and Vegetable Stir-Fry with Buckwheat Noodles:

## Ingredients

1 cup cooked buckwheat noodles

1 cup cooked ground turkey

2 cups mixed vegetables (bell peppers, broccoli, carrots, etc.)

2 tablespoons low-sodium soy sauce

1 tablespoon hoisin sauce

1 tablespoon vegetable oil

1 clove garlic (minced)

1/2 teaspoon grated ginger

Crushed red pepper flakes (optional for added heat)

**How To Prepare**

In a large skillet or wok, heat vegetable oil over medium-high heat.

Add minced garlic and grated ginger, sautéing for a minute until fragrant.

Add the cooked ground turkey and stir-fry for a few minutes until heated through.

Toss in the mixed vegetables and continue stir-frying until they are tender-crisp.

Mix in low-sodium soy sauce and hoisin sauce, ensuring everything is coated with the sauce.

Optionally, add crushed red pepper flakes for added spice.

Serve the turkey and vegetable stir-fry over cooked buckwheat noodles.

**Lentil and Vegetable Curry:**

**Ingredients**

1 cup cooked green or brown lentils

2 cups mixed vegetables (carrots, cauliflower, bell peppers, etc.)

1 can (14 ounces) coconut milk

2 tablespoons curry powder

1 tablespoon vegetable oil

1 small onion (chopped)

2 cloves garlic (minced)

1 teaspoon grated ginger

Salt and pepper to taste

Fresh cilantro for garnish

Cooked basmati rice or naan bread for serving

**How To Prepare**

In a large skillet or pot, heat vegetable oil over medium heat.

Add chopped onion, minced garlic, and grated ginger, sautéing until the onion becomes translucent.

Add the mixed vegetables and cook until they begin to soften.

Stir in the cooked lentils and curry powder, coating everything evenly.

Pour in the coconut milk and simmer for about 10-15 minutes until the vegetables are tender and the flavors meld together.

Season with salt and pepper to taste.

Serve the lentil and vegetable curry over cooked basmati rice or with naan bread.

Garnish with fresh cilantro for added freshness.

**Baked Salmon with Quinoa and Steamed Broccoli:**

**Ingredients**

4 salmon fillets

1 cup quinoa

2 cups vegetable broth or water

2 cups broccoli florets

2 tablespoons olive oil

Lemon wedges for garnish

Fresh dill (optional for garnish)

Salt and pepper to taste

**How To Prepare**

Preheat the oven to 375°F (190°C).

In a baking dish, place the salmon fillets and drizzle with olive oil.

Season with salt and pepper.

Bake the salmon in the preheated oven for about 15-20 minutes or until it's cooked through.

In a saucepan, bring the vegetable broth or water to a boil and add the quinoa.

Reduce the heat, cover, and simmer for about 15 minutes or until the quinoa is cooked and fluffy.

Steam the broccoli until tender-crisp.

Serve the baked salmon alongside cooked quinoa and steamed broccoli.

Garnish with lemon wedges and fresh dill, if desired.

## Baked Chicken with Sweet Potato and Brussels Sprouts:

### Ingredients

4 bone-in, skin-on chicken thighs

2 cups cubed sweet potatoes

2 cups halved Brussels sprouts

2 tablespoons olive oil

1 teaspoon dried thyme

Salt and pepper to taste

### How To Prepare

Preheat the oven to 425°F (220°C).

Place the chicken thighs, sweet potato cubes, and halved Brussels sprouts on a baking sheet lined with parchment paper.

Drizzle olive oil over the chicken and vegetables.

Season with dried thyme, salt, and pepper.

Bake in the preheated oven for about 25-30 minutes or until the chicken is cooked through and the vegetables are tender.

Serve the baked chicken thighs with sweet potato and Brussels sprouts.

**Zucchini Noodles with Pesto and Grilled Chicken:**

**Ingredients**

2 medium zucchini (spiralized into noodles)

4 ounces grilled chicken breast (cooked and sliced)

1/2 cup basil pesto (homemade or store-bought)

Cherry tomatoes for garnish

Grated Parmesan cheese (optional for topping)

**How To Prepare**

In a large skillet, heat the basil pesto over medium heat.

Add the zucchini noodles and toss them in the pesto until they are coated and slightly softened.

Top the zucchini noodles with sliced grilled chicken.

Garnish with cherry tomatoes and optionally, sprinkle grated Parmesan cheese on top.

**Quinoa and Black Bean Buddha Bowl:**

**Ingredients**

1 cup cooked quinoa

1 cup cooked black beans

1 cup diced cucumber

1 cup cherry tomatoes (halved)

1/4 cup diced red onion

2 tablespoons chopped fresh cilantro

2 tablespoons lime juice

2 tablespoons olive oil

Salt and pepper to taste

Avocado slices for garnish

**How To Prepare**

In a large bowl, combine cooked quinoa, cooked black beans, diced cucumber, halved cherry tomatoes, diced red onion, and chopped fresh cilantro.

In a separate small bowl, whisk together lime juice, olive oil, salt, and pepper to make the dressing.

Drizzle the dressing over the quinoa and black bean mixture and toss gently to coat.

Serve the quinoa and black bean Buddha bowl with avocado slices on top.

**Stir-Fried Tofu with Broccoli and Cashews:**

**Ingredients**

1 cup cubed tofu

2 cups broccoli florets

1/2 cup roasted cashews

2 tablespoons low-sodium soy sauce

1 tablespoon hoisin sauce

1 tablespoon vegetable oil

1 clove garlic (minced)

1/2 teaspoon grated ginger

Crushed red pepper flakes (optional for added heat)

Cooked brown rice for serving

**How To Prepare**

In a large skillet or wok, heat vegetable oil over medium-high heat.

Add minced garlic and grated ginger, sautéing for a minute until fragrant.

Add the cubed tofu and stir-fry until it becomes lightly browned.

Toss in the broccoli florets and continue stir-frying until they are tender-crisp.

Mix in low-sodium soy sauce and hoisin sauce, ensuring everything is coated with the sauce.

Add roasted cashews and optionally, crushed red pepper flakes for added spice.

Serve the stir-fried tofu with broccoli and cashews over cooked brown rice.

**Baked Eggplant Parmesan with Mixed Greens Salad:**

**Ingredients**

1 large eggplant (sliced into rounds)

1 cup marinara sauce (homemade or store-bought)

1 cup shredded mozzarella cheese

1/2 cup grated Parmesan cheese

Fresh basil for garnish

Mixed greens salad (arugula, spinach, etc.) with balsamic vinaigrette dressing for serving

**How To Prepare**

Preheat the oven to 375°F (190°C).

Arrange the eggplant rounds on a baking sheet lined with parchment paper.

Spread marinara sauce over each eggplant round.

Sprinkle shredded mozzarella cheese and grated Parmesan cheese on top.

Bake in the preheated oven for about 20-25 minutes or until the cheese is melted and bubbly, and the eggplant is tender.

Garnish with fresh basil.

Serve the baked eggplant Parmesan with a side of mixed greens salad dressed with balsamic vinaigrette.

# BREAST CANCER SOUP RECIPES

**Mushroom Barley Soup:**

**Ingredients**

1 cup pearl barley

4 cups vegetable broth

2 cups sliced mushrooms (cremini or button mushrooms)

1 cup diced carrots

1 cup diced celery

1 small onion (chopped)

2 cloves garlic (minced)

2 tablespoons olive oil

1 teaspoon dried thyme

Salt and pepper to taste


**How To Prepare**

In a large pot, heat olive oil over medium heat.

Add chopped onion and minced garlic, sautéing until the onion becomes translucent.

Stir in the sliced mushrooms, diced carrots, and diced celery, and cook until they begin to soften.

Add the pearl barley and vegetable broth to the pot.

Bring the soup to a boil, then reduce the heat to low, cover, and simmer for about 40-45 minutes or until the barley is cooked and tender.

Stir in dried thyme, salt, and pepper to taste.

Serve the mushroom barley soup hot.

**Minestrone Soup:**

**Ingredients**

1 cup cooked small pasta (such as elbow or ditalini)

4 cups vegetable broth

1 can (14 ounces) diced tomatoes

1 cup diced carrots

1 cup diced celery

1 cup chopped green beans

1 cup cooked kidney beans (drained and rinsed)

1 small onion (chopped)

2 cloves garlic (minced)

2 tablespoons olive oil

1 teaspoon dried oregano

1 teaspoon dried basil

Salt and pepper to taste

## How To Prepare

In a large pot, heat olive oil over medium heat.

Add chopped onion and minced garlic, sautéing until the onion becomes translucent.

Stir in the diced tomatoes, vegetable broth, diced carrots, diced celery, chopped green beans, and cooked kidney beans.

Bring the soup to a boil, then reduce the heat to low, cover, and simmer for about 15-20 minutes or until the vegetables are tender.

Stir in cooked small pasta, dried oregano, dried basil, salt, and pepper to taste.

Serve the minestrone soup hot.

**Carrot Ginger Soup:**

**Ingredients**

4 cups diced carrots

1 small onion (chopped)

2 cloves garlic (minced)

2 tablespoons grated fresh ginger

4 cups vegetable broth

1 cup coconut milk (or any plant-based milk)

2 tablespoons olive oil

Salt and pepper to taste

**How To Prepare**

In a large pot, heat olive oil over medium heat.

Add chopped onion and minced garlic, sautéing until the onion becomes translucent.

Stir in grated fresh ginger and diced carrots, and cook for a few minutes until the carrots begin to soften.

Pour in the vegetable broth and bring the soup to a simmer.

Cook until the carrots are fully tender.

Use an immersion blender or transfer the mixture to a blender and blend until smooth.

Return the blended soup to the pot and stir in the coconut milk.

Season with salt and pepper to taste.

Serve the carrot ginger soup hot.

**Spinach and Chickpea Soup:**

**Ingredients**

1 can (14 ounces) chickpeas (drained and rinsed)

4 cups vegetable broth

2 cups fresh spinach leaves

1 cup diced carrots

1 cup diced celery

1 small onion (chopped)

2 cloves garlic (minced)

2 tablespoons olive oil

1 teaspoon dried thyme

Salt and pepper to taste


**How To Prepare**

In a large pot, heat olive oil over medium heat.

Add chopped onion and minced garlic, sautéing until the onion becomes translucent.

Stir in diced carrots and diced celery, and cook for a few minutes until they begin to soften.

Add the drained chickpeas and vegetable broth to the pot.

Bring the soup to a boil, then reduce the heat to low, cover, and simmer for about 15-20 minutes or until the vegetables are tender.

Stir in fresh spinach leaves and dried thyme, and cook until the spinach wilts.

Season with salt and pepper to taste.

Serve the spinach and chickpea soup hot.

**Turmeric Cauliflower Soup:**

**Ingredients**

1 small head cauliflower (cut into florets)

1 small onion (chopped)

2 cloves garlic (minced)

4 cups vegetable broth

1 cup coconut milk (or any plant-based milk)

2 tablespoons olive oil

1 teaspoon ground turmeric

1/2 teaspoon ground cumin

Salt and pepper to taste

**How To Prepare**

In a large pot, heat olive oil over medium heat.

Add chopped onion and minced garlic, sautéing until the onion becomes translucent.

Stir in cauliflower florets and cook for a few minutes until they begin to soften.

Pour in the vegetable broth and bring the soup to a simmer.

Cook until the cauliflower is fully tender.

Use an immersion blender or transfer the mixture to a blender and blend until smooth.

Return the blended soup to the pot and stir in the coconut milk.

Season with ground turmeric, ground cumin, salt, and pepper to taste.

Serve the turmeric cauliflower soup hot.

**Tomato Basil Soup:**

**Ingredients**

1 can (28 ounces) crushed tomatoes

1 cup vegetable broth

1/2 cup chopped fresh basil leaves

1/4 cup diced onion

2 cloves garlic (minced)

2 tablespoons olive oil

1 tablespoon balsamic vinegar

Salt and pepper to taste


**How To Prepare**

In a large pot, heat olive oil over medium heat.

Add diced onion and minced garlic, sautéing until the onion becomes translucent.

Stir in the crushed tomatoes, vegetable broth, and chopped basil leaves.

Bring the soup to a simmer and cook for about 15-20 minutes to let the flavors meld together.

Stir in balsamic vinegar and season with salt and pepper to taste.

Serve the tomato basil soup hot.

**Thai Coconut Curry Soup with Shrimp:**

**Ingredients**

1 pound shrimp (peeled and deveined)

4 cups vegetable broth

1 can (14 ounces) coconut milk

1 cup sliced mushrooms (cremini or button mushrooms)

1 cup sliced bell peppers (any color)

2 cloves garlic (minced)

2 tablespoons red curry paste

1 tablespoon vegetable oil

1 tablespoon soy sauce

1 tablespoon lime juice

Fresh cilantro for garnish

Cooked rice noodles for serving

## How To Prepare

In a large pot, heat vegetable oil over medium heat.

Add minced garlic and sauté until fragrant.

Stir in red curry paste and cook for a minute to release its flavors.

Pour in the vegetable broth and coconut milk, and bring the soup to a simmer.

Add sliced mushrooms and sliced bell peppers to the pot, and cook until they are tender.

Stir in peeled and deveined shrimp, and cook until they turn pink and are fully cooked.

Mix in soy sauce and lime juice to add some tangy and savory flavors.

Serve the Thai coconut curry soup with shrimp over cooked rice noodles.

Garnish with fresh cilantro for added freshness.

**Butternut Squash Soup:**

**Ingredients**

1 medium butternut squash (peeled, seeded, and cubed)

1 small onion (chopped)

2 cloves garlic (minced)

4 cups vegetable broth

1 cup coconut milk (or any plant-based milk)

2 tablespoons olive oil

1 teaspoon ground cinnamon

Salt and pepper to taste

**How To Prepare**

Preheat the oven to 400°F (200°C).

Toss the cubed butternut squash with 1 tablespoon of olive oil, ground cinnamon, salt, and pepper.

Spread the seasoned butternut squash on a baking sheet lined with parchment paper.

Roast in the preheated oven for about 25-30 minutes or until the squash is tender and slightly caramelized.

In a large pot, heat 1 tablespoon of olive oil over medium heat.

Add chopped onion and minced garlic, sautéing until the onion becomes translucent.

Stir in the roasted butternut squash and vegetable broth.

Bring the soup to a simmer and cook for a few minutes.

Use an immersion blender or transfer the mixture to a blender and blend until smooth.

Return the blended soup to the pot and stir in the coconut milk.

Season with salt and pepper to taste.

Serve the creamy butternut squash soup hot.

**Quinoa Vegetable Soup:**

**Ingredients**

1 cup cooked quinoa

4 cups vegetable broth

1 cup diced carrots

1 cup diced celery

1 cup diced zucchini

1 small onion (chopped)

2 cloves garlic (minced)

2 tablespoons olive oil

1 teaspoon dried thyme

Salt and pepper to taste

## How To Prepare

In a large pot, heat olive oil over medium heat.

Add chopped onion and minced garlic, sautéing until the onion becomes translucent.

Stir in diced carrots, diced celery, and diced zucchini, and cook for a few minutes until they begin to soften.

Pour in the vegetable broth and bring the soup to a simmer.

Cook until the vegetables are fully tender.

Stir in the cooked quinoa and dried thyme, and simmer for a few more minutes.

Season with salt and pepper to taste.

Serve the quinoa vegetable soup hot.

**Creamy Broccoli Soup:**

**Ingredients**

4 cups chopped broccoli florets

1 small onion (chopped)

2 cloves garlic (minced)

3 cups vegetable broth

1 cup unsweetened almond milk (or any plant-based milk)

2 tablespoons olive oil

Salt and pepper to taste

**How To Prepare**

In a large pot, heat olive oil over medium heat.

Add chopped onion and minced garlic, sautéing until the onion becomes translucent.

Add chopped broccoli florets and cook for a few minutes until slightly tender.

Pour in the vegetable broth and bring the mixture to a simmer.

Cook until the broccoli is fully tender.

Use an immersion blender or transfer the mixture to a blender and blend until smooth.

Return the blended soup to the pot and stir in the almond milk.

Season with salt and pepper to taste.

Serve the creamy broccoli soup hot.

**Red Lentil and Spinach Soup:**

**Ingredients**

1 cup red lentils

4 cups vegetable broth

2 cups fresh spinach leaves

1 cup diced carrots

1 cup diced celery

1 small onion (chopped)

2 cloves garlic (minced)

2 tablespoons olive oil

1 teaspoon ground cumin

Salt and pepper to taste


**How To Prepare**

In a large pot, heat olive oil over medium heat.

Add chopped onion and minced garlic, sautéing until the onion becomes translucent.

Stir in diced carrots and diced celery, and cook for a few minutes until they begin to soften.

Add red lentils and vegetable broth to the pot.

Bring the soup to a boil, then reduce the heat to low, cover, and simmer for about 15-20 minutes or until the lentils are fully cooked and tender.

Stir in fresh spinach leaves and ground cumin, and cook until the spinach wilts.

Season with salt and pepper to taste.

Serve the red lentil and spinach soup hot.

**Sweet Potato and Black Bean Soup:**

**Ingredients**

2 cups cubed sweet potatoes

1 can (14 ounces) black beans (drained and rinsed)

4 cups vegetable broth

1 cup diced tomatoes

1 small onion (chopped)

2 cloves garlic (minced)

2 tablespoons olive oil

1 teaspoon ground cumin

1/2 teaspoon chili powder

Salt and pepper to taste

**How To Prepare**

In a large pot, heat olive oil over medium heat.

Add chopped onion and minced garlic, sautéing until the onion becomes translucent.

Stir in cubed sweet potatoes, diced tomatoes, and black beans, and cook for a few minutes until the sweet potatoes start to soften.

Pour in the vegetable broth and bring the soup to a simmer.

Cook until the sweet potatoes are fully tender.

Mix in ground cumin, chili powder, salt, and pepper to taste.

Serve the sweet potato and black bean soup hot.

**Chicken and Vegetable Soup:**

**Ingredients**

1 pound boneless, skinless chicken breasts (cooked and shredded)

4 cups chicken broth

1 cup mixed vegetables (carrots, celery, onions, etc.)

1/2 cup diced tomatoes

2 cloves garlic (minced)

2 tablespoons olive oil

1 teaspoon dried thyme

Salt and pepper to taste

**How To Prepare**

In a large pot, heat olive oil over medium heat.

Add minced garlic and sauté until fragrant.

Add the mixed vegetables and cook until they begin to soften.

Stir in the shredded cooked chicken, chicken broth, diced tomatoes (with their juice), and dried thyme.

Bring the soup to a boil, then reduce the heat to low, cover, and simmer for about 15-20 minutes to let the flavors meld together.

Season with salt and pepper to taste.

Serve the chicken and vegetable soup hot.

**Miso Soup with Tofu and Seaweed:**

**Ingredients**

4 cups vegetable broth

1/4 cup miso paste

1/2 cup cubed tofu

1/4 cup sliced green onions

1 sheet dried seaweed (nori) cut into thin strips

1 tablespoon soy sauce

1 tablespoon rice vinegar

1 teaspoon sesame oil

## How To Prepare

In a large pot, heat vegetable broth over medium heat.

In a small bowl, dissolve miso paste in a bit of warm water to create a smooth paste.

Add the miso paste to the vegetable broth and stir to combine.

Stir in cubed tofu, sliced green onions, and dried seaweed.

Let the soup simmer for a few minutes to allow the flavors to meld together.

Mix in soy sauce, rice vinegar, and sesame oil to add depth and savory taste.

Serve the miso soup with tofu and seaweed hot.

**Roasted Red Pepper and Tomato Soup:**

**Ingredients**

2 large red bell peppers

1 can (28 ounces) crushed tomatoes

4 cups vegetable broth

1 small onion (chopped)

2 cloves garlic (minced)

2 tablespoons olive oil

1 teaspoon dried basil

1/2 teaspoon smoked paprika

Salt and pepper to taste

## How To Prepare

Preheat the oven to 400°F (200°C).

Cut the red bell peppers in half and remove the seeds and stems.

Place the pepper halves on a baking sheet lined with parchment paper, cut-side down.

Roast the red bell peppers in the preheated oven for about 20-25 minutes or until the skin becomes charred and blistered.

Remove the peppers from the oven and let them cool. Then peel off the skin and roughly chop the peppers.

In a large pot, heat olive oil over medium heat.

Add chopped onion and minced garlic, sautéing until the onion becomes translucent.

Stir in the crushed tomatoes, roasted red peppers, and vegetable broth.

Bring the soup to a simmer, then reduce the heat to low and cook for about 15-20 minutes.

Stir in dried basil, smoked paprika, salt, and pepper to taste.

Use an immersion blender or transfer the mixture to a blender and blend until smooth.

Return the blended soup to the pot and let it simmer for a few more minutes.

Serve the roasted red pepper and tomato soup hot.

# BREAST CANCER DESSERT RECIPES

**Chocolate Avocado Mousse:**

**Ingredients**

2 ripe avocados

1/4 cup cocoa powder

1/4 cup maple syrup (or honey)

1 teaspoon vanilla extract

Pinch of salt

Fresh berries for garnish (optional)

**How To Prepare**

In a food processor or blender, blend together avocados, cocoa powder, maple syrup (or honey), vanilla extract, and a pinch of salt until smooth and creamy.

Taste and adjust sweetness if needed.

Scoop the chocolate avocado mousse into serving bowls or glasses.

Optionally, garnish with fresh berries on top.

Refrigerate for at least 30 minutes before serving to allow the mousse to chill and set.

**Banana-Oatmeal Cookies:**

**Ingredients**

2 ripe bananas (mashed)

1 cup rolled oats

1/4 cup raisins (or chocolate chips)

1/4 cup chopped nuts (such as walnuts or almonds)

1 teaspoon vanilla extract

**How To Prepare**

Preheat the oven to 350°F (175°C) and line a baking sheet with parchment paper.

In a bowl, mix mashed bananas, rolled oats, raisins (or chocolate chips), chopped nuts, and vanilla extract until well combined.

Drop spoonfuls of the cookie mixture onto the prepared baking sheet.

Flatten each cookie slightly with the back of a spoon.

Bake for about 15-18 minutes or until the cookies are golden brown.

Let the cookies cool on a wire rack before serving.

**Almond Butter and Berry Rice Cakes:**

**Ingredients**

4 rice cakes

1/4 cup almond butter (or any nut butter)

Fresh berries of your choice (such as raspberries, blueberries, etc.)

**How To Prepare**

Spread almond butter (or any nut butter) over each rice cake.

Top the almond butter with fresh berries.

Enjoy these light and satisfying rice cake desserts.

**Lemon Poppy Seed Muffins (using whole grain flour):**

**Ingredients**

1 cup whole grain flour

1/4 cup almond flour (or any nut flour)

1/4 cup maple syrup (or honey)

1/4 cup plain Greek yogurt

1/4 cup unsweetened applesauce

1/4 cup fresh lemon juice

1 tablespoon poppy seeds

1 teaspoon baking powder

1/2 teaspoon baking soda

Zest of 1 lemon

Pinch of salt

**How To Prepare**

Preheat the oven to 350°F (175°C) and line a muffin tin with paper liners.

In a bowl, whisk together whole grain flour, almond flour, baking powder, baking soda, poppy seeds, lemon zest, and a pinch of salt.

In a separate bowl, mix maple syrup (or honey), Greek yogurt, unsweetened applesauce, and fresh lemon juice.

Combine the wet ingredients with the dry ingredients and stir until just combined.

Scoop the muffin batter into the prepared muffin tin.

Bake for about 18-20 minutes or until a toothpick inserted into the center of a muffin comes out clean.

Let the muffins cool in the tin for a few minutes before transferring them to a wire rack to cool completely.

**Coconut Milk Panna Cotta with Berries:**

**Ingredients**

1 can (14 ounces) coconut milk (full fat)

1/4 cup maple syrup (or honey)

1 teaspoon vanilla extract

2 teaspoons agar agar powder (or gelatin for non-vegan option)

Fresh berries for topping (such as strawberries, blueberries, etc.)

**How To Prepare**

In a saucepan, whisk together coconut milk, maple syrup (or honey), and vanilla extract.

Sprinkle agar agar powder (or gelatin) over the mixture and let it sit for a minute.

Heat the mixture over medium heat, stirring constantly, until it comes to a gentle boil.

Reduce the heat to low and simmer for 2 minutes to allow the agar agar (or gelatin) to dissolve completely.

Remove the saucepan from the heat and let the mixture cool slightly.

Pour the coconut milk mixture into individual serving glasses or molds.

Refrigerate for at least 2 hours or until the panna cotta sets.

Before serving, top the panna cotta with fresh berries.

**Pumpkin Spice Energy Bites:**

**Ingredients**

1 cup rolled oats

1/2 cup pumpkin puree

1/4 cup almond butter (or any nut butter)

1/4 cup maple syrup (or honey)

1 teaspoon pumpkin pie spice

1/2 teaspoon vanilla extract

1/4 cup unsweetened shredded coconut (optional, for coating)

**How To Prepare**

In a bowl, mix rolled oats, pumpkin puree, almond butter (or any nut butter), maple syrup (or honey), pumpkin pie spice, and vanilla extract until well combined.

Refrigerate the mixture for 15-30 minutes to make it easier to handle.

After chilling, take small portions of the mixture and roll them into bite-sized balls.

Optionally, roll the energy bites in unsweetened shredded coconut for extra texture and flavor.

Store the pumpkin spice energy bites in an airtight container in the refrigerator until serving.

**Mixed Berry Parfait:**

**Ingredients**

1 cup mixed berries (strawberries, blueberries, raspberries, etc.)

1 cup Greek yogurt (plain or flavored)

1/4 cup granola

1 tablespoon honey (optional)

**How To Prepare**

In a serving glass or bowl, layer the mixed berries, Greek yogurt, and granola.

Optionally, drizzle honey over the top for added sweetness.

Repeat the layering until you fill the glass or bowl.

Serve the mixed berry parfait chilled.

**Greek Yogurt with Honey and Almonds:**

**Ingredients**

1 cup Greek yogurt (plain or flavored)

1 tablespoon honey

2 tablespoons sliced almonds

**How To Prepare**

In a bowl, scoop the Greek yogurt.

Drizzle honey over the top and sprinkle sliced almonds.

Mix lightly and enjoy the creamy and sweet yogurt dessert.

**Strawberry Frozen Yogurt:**

**Ingredients**

2 cups frozen strawberries

1 cup plain Greek yogurt

2 tablespoons honey (or maple syrup)

1 teaspoon vanilla extract

**How To Prepare**

In a blender or food processor, blend frozen strawberries, Greek yogurt, honey (or maple syrup), and vanilla extract until smooth and creamy.

Taste and adjust sweetness if needed.

Pour the strawberry frozen yogurt into a shallow dish and freeze for at least 2 hours or until firm.

Before serving, let the frozen yogurt sit at room temperature for a few minutes to soften slightly.

Scoop the strawberry frozen yogurt into serving bowls and enjoy this refreshing treat.

**Blueberry Almond Crisp (using whole grain oats):**

**Ingredients**

2 cups fresh blueberries

1 tablespoon lemon juice

1/4 cup maple syrup (or honey)

1/2 cup whole grain oats

1/4 cup almond flour (or any nut flour)

1/4 cup sliced almonds

2 tablespoons coconut oil (or butter)

Pinch of salt


**How To Prepare**

Preheat the oven to 350°F (175°C) and grease a baking dish.

In a bowl, toss fresh blueberries with lemon juice and maple syrup (or honey).

In a separate bowl, mix whole grain oats, almond flour (or any nut flour), sliced almonds, coconut oil (or butter), and a pinch of salt until crumbly.

Spread the blueberry mixture in the greased baking dish.

Sprinkle the oat-almond topping over the blueberries.

Bake for about 25-30 minutes or until the topping is golden brown and the blueberries are bubbly.

Let the blueberry almond crisp cool slightly before serving.

**Chocolate-Dipped Strawberries:**

**Ingredients**

Fresh strawberries (washed and dried)

1/2 cup dark chocolate chips (or any chocolate of your choice)

1 teaspoon coconut oil

**How To Prepare**

In a microwave-safe bowl, melt the dark chocolate chips (or any chocolate of your choice) with coconut oil in the microwave, stirring every 15-20 seconds until smooth.

Dip each strawberry into the melted chocolate, coating them halfway.

Place the chocolate-dipped strawberries on a parchment-lined tray.

Refrigerate the strawberries for a few minutes to allow the chocolate to harden.

Serve the chocolate-dipped strawberries chilled.

**Baked Apples with Cinnamon and Walnuts:**

**Ingredients**

4 medium apples (such as Granny Smith or Honeycrisp)

1 tablespoon melted coconut oil (or butter)

1 tablespoon maple syrup (or honey)

1 teaspoon ground cinnamon

1/4 cup chopped walnuts

**How To Prepare**

Preheat the oven to 375°F (190°C).

Core the apples and remove some of the flesh to create space for the filling.

In a small bowl, mix melted coconut oil (or butter), maple syrup (or honey), and ground cinnamon.

Brush the mixture over the apples, coating them evenly.

Place the apples in a baking dish and fill each with chopped walnuts.

Cover the baking dish with aluminum foil and bake for about 25-30 minutes or until the apples are tender.

Serve the baked apples warm.

**Mango Sorbet:**

## Ingredients

2 cups frozen mango chunks

1/4 cup coconut milk (or any plant-based milk)

1 tablespoon honey (or maple syrup)

1 teaspoon lime juice

## How To Prepare

In a blender or food processor, blend frozen mango chunks, coconut milk (or any plant-based milk), honey (or maple syrup), and lime juice until smooth and creamy.

Taste and adjust sweetness if needed.

Pour the mango sorbet mixture into a shallow dish and freeze for at least 2 hours or until firm.

Before serving, let the sorbet sit at room temperature for a few minutes to soften slightly.

Scoop the mango sorbet into serving bowls and enjoy this tropical delight.

**Carrot Cake Energy Balls:**

**Ingredients**

1 cup shredded carrots

1 cup rolled oats

1/2 cup almond butter (or any nut butter)

1/4 cup maple syrup (or honey)

1/4 cup chopped walnuts

1 teaspoon ground cinnamon

1/2 teaspoon ground ginger

Pinch of nutmeg

**How To Prepare**

In a bowl, mix shredded carrots, rolled oats, almond butter (or any nut butter), maple syrup (or honey), chopped walnuts, ground cinnamon, ground ginger, and a pinch of nutmeg until well combined.

Refrigerate the mixture for 15-30 minutes to make it easier to handle.

After chilling, take small portions of the mixture and roll them into bite-sized balls.

Store the carrot cake energy balls in an airtight container in the refrigerator until serving.

**Chia Seed Pudding with Fresh Fruit:**

**Ingredients**

1/4 cup chia seeds

1 cup almond milk (or any plant-based milk)

1 tablespoon maple syrup (or honey)

1/2 teaspoon vanilla extract

Fresh fruit of your choice (such as sliced strawberries, blueberries, etc.)

**How To Prepare**

In a bowl, whisk together chia seeds, almond milk, maple syrup, and vanilla extract.

Let the mixture sit for 5 minutes, then whisk again to avoid clumps.

Cover the bowl and refrigerate the chia seed pudding overnight or for at least 2 hours until it thickens.

Before serving, top the chia seed pudding with fresh fruit.

# CHAPTER IV: FINAL NOTES

As we reach the conclusion of this cookbook, we embark on a collective journey inspired by the principles of wholesome nutrition, self-sufficiency, and unwavering optimism. Our aspiration extends beyond merely providing a practical resource for those battling breast cancer; we envision the recipes, guidance, and anecdotes shared within these pages as catalysts for profound transformation.

Throughout this culinary exploration, we've delved into the intricate interplay between food and health, recognizing the pivotal role nutrition plays in resilience amid adversity. This cookbook serves as a testament to the empowering potential inherent in conscientious nourishment of both body and spirit. It's a celebration of the revitalizing essence of mindful eating, fostering a deep sense of self-care and compassion.

Beyond its culinary offerings, this cookbook serves as a poignant reminder of your inherent strength, resilience, and capacity for healing. It transcends its role as a mere culinary guide, inviting you to embrace each dish as a gesture of self-love and affirmation. Whether indulging in a nourishing meal, cultivating mindfulness, or expressing creativity through culinary artistry, every step taken is a stride toward personal growth and fulfillment.

May these dishes and rituals serve as beacons of solace, motivation, and restoration on your journey. As you partake in the aromatic herbs and spices, may they evoke a sense of vitality within you. As you savor each dish, may it replenish your inner reservoirs of strength and resilience. And as you apply the cooking techniques, may you find moments of serenity and renewal amidst life's challenges.

Our sincerest wish is for you to embrace the journey ahead with unwavering strength, courage, and the firm belief in your ability to shape your destiny. As you navigate the trials of breast cancer treatment, may this cookbook stand as a steadfast source of encouragement, empowering you to face each day with dignity, fortitude, and an appreciation for the profound beauty inherent in life's transformative journey.